DASH DIET
Pressure Cooker
COOKBOOK

**Easy and Delicious DASH Diet Pressure Cooker Recipes
For Weight Loss, Energy, and Vibrant Health**

Copyright © 2016 Anne Gibson

All Rights Reserved.

Published by The Fruitful Mind

www.fruitfulbooks.com

Disclaimer

TABLE OF CONTENTS

Introduction

Grains, vegetables, fruits, low-fat dairy products, seeds, nuts, and lean meat all form the base of the DASH diet. So, there are no strict restrictions, only amazing benefits. Besides giving you a way of turning to healthy eating habits, the DASH diet is primarily known for showing great results in lowering high blood pressure. This diet is rich in several minerals like calcium, zinc, iron, manganese, and potassium, and these nutrients primarily help to regulate the blood pressure. Also, the diet is low in saturated fat and cholesterol but provides a significant amount of protein, which can also help people suffering from high blood pressure.

The DASH diet is also known for its heart health benefits because it decreases the bad cholesterol while at the same time it increases the good cholesterol. Also, there have been studies showing that the DASH diet can help people suffering from diabetes control this condition.

Knowing what kind of foods make the foundation of this diet makes it clear that it can also be used to lose weight and excess fat. Following this kind of diet means losing about 500 calories a day. Combine that with exercise, and you will get slim fast. What supports this is also the fact that the DASH diet, rich in protein and fiber, keeps you full for a longer time and thus prevents overeating and gaining weight.

The DASH diet is one of the few diets that can help you meet your daily requirement for potassium, which, besides countering the effect of salt to raise blood pressure, also helps in preventing osteoporosis. This diet also provides sufficient amounts of vitamin B 12, calcium, and fiber, which are required for proper cell metabolism, building and maintaining strong bones, keeping blood sugar levels stable, and preventing obesity.

And now let's move to pressure cooking. Although pressure cookers are praised for preparing meals very fast, their most important benefit is something else. Foods we use in preparing meals contain water-soluble vitamins, such as vitamin C and vitamins of the B complex. When you cook your food in large quantities of water, as you do with boiling, these vitamins get washed away. With pressure cookers, not only will you use less amount of water to cook your vegetables, but there is also no way that anything can escape from the pressure cooker. So, all the nutrients in the food you prepare in the pressure cooker remain there.

In this book, you will find recipes that combine these two ways of healthy eating to get fully nutritious and delicious meals. The recipes are organized into groups of chicken, beef, pork, seafood/fish, and vegetarian recipes. Just pick what you would like to eat, go there and choose the recipe you want to prepare. No matter which one you choose, you will surely prepare an amazing surprise for your family members' taste buds.

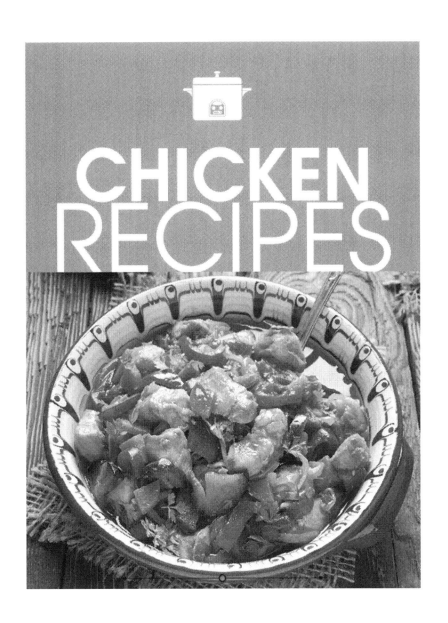

CHICKEN RECIPES

Acapulco Chicken

Calories: 400

Fats: 8g

Carbs: 67g

Protein: 17g

Sodium: 75g

Servings: 6

Cook time: 15 minutes

Ingredients:

½ cup raisins

1 ½ cup orange juice

½ cup orange marmalade

1 teaspoon ground cinnamon

4 tablespoons brown sugar

1 cup rice

½ teaspoon freshly grated ginger

2 tablespoons olive oil

3 thick, boneless, skinless chicken breast halves, cut into 1-inch pieces

½ cup flaked coconut

Salt and pepper

Directions:

Combine the raisins, orange juice, and marmalade in a saucepan. Place over medium heat and heat until the marmalade melts. Remove the saucepan from the heat and mix in the cinnamon, brown sugar, rice, and ginger. Set aside.

Pour the olive oil in a pressure cooker, and when the oil is hot enough, add the chicken chunks. Leave the chicken to brown lightly and then add the orange mixture.

Close and lock the lid of your pressure cooker. Cook on high pressure for 10 minutes. When the cooking time is up, use the quick release method to release pressure.

Open the pressure cooker, season with pepper and salt and mix in the coconut flakes. Serve warm.

Spanish-Style Pressure Cooker Chicken

Calories: 375

Fats: 6g

Carbs: 58g

Protein: 17g

Sodium: 75g

Servings: 4

Cook time: 10 minutes

Ingredients:

1 tablespoon canola oil

2 large onions, chopped

1 pound boneless, skinless chicken breasts, cut into ½-inch pieces

1 sweet red pepper, thinly sliced

8 garlic cloves, minced

6 tomatoes, diced

1 mild chili pepper, seeded and finely chopped

1/2 cup raisins

1 stick cinnamon

1/4 teaspoon crushed red pepper flakes

8 corn tortillas, warmed

Directions:

Pour the oil in your pressure cooker, and when it is hot enough, add the chicken, garlic, and onions and sauté over medium heat. When the chicken is lightly browned, mix in the raisins, tomatoes, sweet peppers, cinnamon and chili peppers.

Close and lock the lid. Cook on high pressure for 5 minutes. When the cooking time is up, leave the pressure to release naturally. This will take about 5-10 minutes.

Open the pressure cooker and discard the cinnamon. Mix in the red pepper flakes and flour. Heat the mixture again for 2-5 minutes until it has thickened a bit. Use the mixture to fill warm tortillas.

Pressure-Cooker Easy Chicken and Rice

Calories: 380

Fats: 8g

Carbs: 55g

Protein: 18g

Sodium: 70g

Servings: 4

Cook time: 20 minutes

Ingredients:

4 (12-ounce) bone-in split chicken breasts, skin removed

1 tablespoon vegetable oil

1 onion, finely chopped

3 carrots, peeled and cut into ½-inch pieces

4 garlic cloves, minced

1 ½ cups long-grain white rice

2 cups low-sodium chicken broth

3 tablespoons minced fresh parsley

1 cup frozen peas

2 teaspoons lemon juice

Directions:

Pat dry the chicken and season it with pepper and salt. Set aside.

Pour the oil in your pressure cooker over medium-high heat. When the oil is hot enough, add the chicken and brown for 6 minutes until golden. When the chicken is done, transfer it to a plate and set aside.

Pour the fat from the pressure cooker leaving only 1 tablespoon. Mix in the onion, carrot, a pinch of salt and sauté for 5 minutes until the vegetables have softened. Add the garlic and rice and cook for half a minute until fragrant.

Pour in the broth and scrape up the browned bits that got stuck to the bottom of the cooker. Add the browned chicken and nestle it into the rice.

Close and lock the lid. Cook on high heat for 15 minutes. When the cooking time is up, release the pressure using the quick release method.

Open the pressure cooker and transfer the chicken to a serving dish. Cover loosely with aluminum foil to keep it warm.

To finish preparing the rice, sprinkle the parsley and peas over the rice. Drizzle with the lemon juice, cover and let stand for 5 minutes. Fluff the rice, season with pepper and salt and serve with the chicken.

Chicken Delirious Rice

Calories: 426

Fats: 3.7g

Carbs: 66g

Protein: 14.7g

Sodium: 71mg

Servings: 8

Cook time: 30 minutes

Ingredients:

2 green bell peppers, chopped

2 onions, chopped

4 carrots, cut into match-stick size pieces

1 pound skinless, boneless chicken breasts, cut into cubes

1 cup lemon juice

1 ½ cup orange juice

¾ cup vinegar

1 cup brown sugar

2 teaspoons ground ginger

1 teaspoon red pepper flakes, or more to taste

1 teaspoon Asian (toasted) sesame oil

2 ½ cups water

1 ¼ cups white rice

1 tablespoon cornstarch

Directions:

Combine the green bell peppers, onions, and carrots in your pressure cooker. Cook for a minute and then add the chicken.

In a bowl, whisk together the lemon juice, 1 cup orange juice, vinegar, brown sugar, ginger, red pepper flakes, and sesame oil in a bowl. Pour this mixture over the chicken. Stir well to coat the chicken with the sauce.

Close and lock the lid of your pressure cooker. Cook on medium pressure for 15 minutes. When the cooking time is up, release the pressure using either the natural method or the quick release method. Keep the chicken warm.

To prepare the rice, combine it with the water in a microwave-safe dish. Cook for about 15 minutes on high until the water has been absorbed.

In a bowl, combine the cornstarch and ½ cup of orange juice and mix well until blended. Add this mixture to the chicken in the pressure cooker. The sauce should thicken. Serve the chicken over a bed of rice.

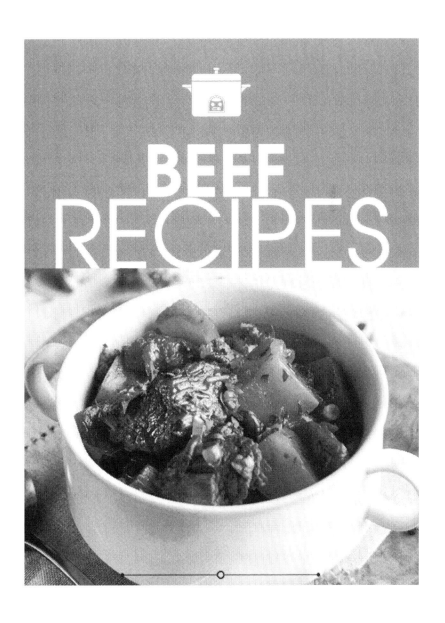

BEEF RECIPES

Easy Beef Stew

Calories: 580.7

Fat: 24.6g

Carbs: 48.3g

Protein: 40.9g

Sodium: 182mg

Serves: 4

Cook time: 35 minutes

Ingredients:

1 1/2 pounds rump roast

1 tablespoon olive oil

2 garlic cloves, chopped

4 carrots, peeled and cut into chunks

1 large onion, cut up

4 potatoes, cut into chunks

4 celery ribs, peeled and cut into chunks

1–2 teaspoons dried parsley

1 ½ - 2 cups water

Black pepper to taste

Directions:

Prepare the roast by cutting it into chunks. These should be 1-inch cubes or larger if you wish.

Pour the oil in your pressure cooker and heat until the oil gets hot. Add the meat chunks to the pressure cooker to sear it. Stir the meat frequently as it browns.

When the meat cubes brown on all sides, stir in the chopped garlic clove. Cook for a minute, stirring constantly. Mix in the carrots, onions, potatoes, celery, and parsley. Season with black pepper and pour in the water.

Close and lock the lid of your pressure cooker. Bring to high pressure over high heat and cook for 15 minutes. When the cooking time is up, release the pressure using the cold water release method (hold your pressure cooker under a · stream of cold water until the pressure releases). Open the cooker and serve immediately.

Beef and Pineapple Medley

Calories: 265

Fat: 0.6g

Carbs: 60g

Protein: 6g

Sodium: 204mg

Serves: 4-6

Cook time: 52 minutes

Ingredients:

1 pound beef, cubed

1½ cups water

2 garlic cloves, finely chopped

1 onion, roughly chopped

1 teaspoon ground ginger

1 pound pineapple, cubed

2 carrots, roughly chopped

2 fresh tomatoes, roughly chopped

2 big potatoes, cubed

1 teaspoon ground oregano

1 whole red pepper, large dice

1 pinch black pepper

Directions:

Add the beef cubes along with the water in your pressure cooker.

Close and lock the lid. Cook at high pressure for 15 minutes. When the cooking time is up, release the pressure using the quick release method (release the pressure using the valve).

Add the garlic clove, onion, and ginger and cook uncovered for 2 minutes. Mix in the remaining ingredients.

Close and lock the lid. Cook on high pressure for 15 more minutes. When the time is up, release the pressure through the valve. Serve warm.

Chili Con Carne

Calories: 270

Fat: 2g

Carbs: 55g

Protein: 7g

Sodium: 190mg

Servings: 4

Cook time: 30 minutes

Ingredients:

4 tablespoons olive oil, divided

1 pound ground beef

2 garlic cloves, finely chopped

1 medium onion, chopped

1 bay leaf

8 tomatoes, peeled and chopped

5 ounces kidney beans, soaked overnight

1 tablespoon chili powder

1/2 teaspoon ground cumin

2/3 cup water

Directions:

Pour one tablespoon of oil into your pressure cooker. When the oil is hot enough, add the ground beef and cook until browned. When done, remove from the cooker.

Pour the remaining oil in the cooker and add the onions and garlic. Stir-fry the onions until lightly browned.

Return the beef to the cooker along with the rest of the ingredients. Stir well to combine everything.

Close and lock the lid. Cook on high pressure for 18 minutes. When the cooking time is up, leave the pressure to release on its own.

Open the pressure cooker, discard the bay leaves and serve the chili hot.

Beef Pot Roast with Gravy

Calories: 264

Fat: 11g

Carbs: 15g

Protein: 23g

Sodium: 180mg

Servings: 2-4

Cook time: 1 hour 10 min

Ingredients:

2 teaspoons olive oil

1 boneless chuck roast, trimmed

¼ teaspoon freshly ground black pepper

3½ cups water

4 thyme sprigs, tied with twine

3 large carrots, peeled and cut into 2-inch pieces

3 large parsnips, peeled and cut into 2-inch pieces

3 garlic cloves, chopped

1 pound Yukon gold potatoes, peeled and diced

1 pound turnips, each cut into 8 wedges

1 large onion, cut into 8 wedges

2 tablespoons all-purpose flour

Directions:

Heat your pressure cooker over medium-high heat. Pour in the oil and swirl to coat.

Season the roast with pepper and salt. Place the seasoned roast into the cooker and sauté for 5 minutes, allowing it to brown on all sides.

Pour in the water. Close and lock the lid. Cook over high pressure for 35 minutes. When the cooking time is up, release the pressure either using the quick or cold water release method.

Once the pressure has released, add the thyme, carrots, parsnips, garlic, turnips, potatoes, and onion.

Close and lock the lid. Return to high pressure and cook for 8 minutes.

Release the pressure again using the cold water or quick pressure release method. Open the cooker and leave to sit for 5 minutes.

Take the roast out of the pressure cooker, slice it thinly and serve on a platter. Using a slotted spoon, remove the vegetables from the cooker and arrange them on the platter with the roast slices. Cover the meat and veggies and keep warm.

Line a sieve with cheesecloth and place it over a large bowl. Pour the cooking liquid into the sieve and strain it into the bowl, discarding solids.

Pour this liquid into a large skillet and bring to the boil. Cook for about 15 minutes until the liquid is reduced to about 1½ cups.

Reserve ¼ cup of the cooking liquid and leave the remaining in the skillet. Add the flour to that 1/4 cup of liquid and mix until it is blended well. Pour this mixture into the skillet and cook for 2 minutes until the mixture has thickened slightly.

Whisk the sauce constantly while cooking. Serve this sauce with the roast slices and veggies.

Beef Chili

Calories: 358

Fat: 25g

Carbs: 15g

Protein: 24g

Sodium: 235mg

Servings: 4-6

Cook time: 35 minutes

Ingredients:

1 tablespoon olive oil

1 pound cubed beef stew meat

1 large clove garlic, minced

1 onion, peeled and chopped

1/4 cup cranberry juice

1/2 cup fat-free reduced-sodium beef broth

2 tablespoons red wine vinegar

1/2 teaspoon dried oregano

1/2 teaspoon dried rosemary

6 whole black peppercorns

1 teaspoon ground cumin

2 bay leaves

1 pinch ground cloves

1/8 teaspoon ground cinnamon

1 1/2 teaspoons light brown sugar

1/4 teaspoon ground black pepper

12 whole plum tomatoes, peeled and cut into 2-inch pieces

1/2 cup water

2 carrots, peeled and sliced

2 potatoes, peeled and diced

Directions:

Pour the olive oil in your pressure cooker over medium-high heat. When the oil is hot enough, add half the beef and cook stirring frequently until the beef is browned on all sides.

When the beef is done, use a slotted spoon to remove it from the pressure cooker. Repeat the same process with the remaining beef and set all aside.

Add the chopped onion to the pressure cooker and cook for a minute, stirring constantly. Mix in the garlic and cook for one minute. Add the cranberry juice, beef broth, and red wine vinegar and mix everything well.

Place the oregano, rosemary, and peppercorns in a mortar and crush them nicely or use a spice grinder. Stir this mixture into the pressure cooker along with cumin, bay leaves, cloves, cinnamon, brown sugar, and black pepper.

Add the potatoes, crushing them to release their juices. Pour in the water as well and mix in the carrots and potatoes.

Return the browned beef to the pressure cooker. If you use a 5-quart pressure cooker, it should be about half full. Cover and lock the lid. Cook over high heat for 15 minutes.

When the cooking time is up, release the pressure using the natural release method. This will take about 10-15 minutes. Check the seasonings and serve warm.

Bangladeshi Beef Curry

Calories: 320

Fats: 23g

Carbs: 8.8g

Protein: 20g

Sodium: 50mg

Servings: 4-6

Cook time: 1h 45 min

Ingredients:

3 tablespoons olive oil

1 onion, chopped

6 cloves garlic, minced

5 green chili peppers, finely sliced

1 teaspoon grated ginger

3 whole cardamom seeds

2 whole cloves

2-inch cinnamon stick

1 teaspoon ground cumin

1 teaspoon ground coriander

1 teaspoon ground turmeric

1 teaspoon garlic powder

1 teaspoon cayenne pepper

1 ½ cups water

2 pounds boneless beef chuck, cut into 1-1/2-inch pieces

Directions:

Pour the oil in a skillet and heat it over medium heat. Add the onion and sauté for about 5 minutes until the onion has softened and turned translucent.

Reduce the heat to medium-low and cook for abou15 to 20 more minutes. Stir frequently. The onion should be very tender and dark brown in color.

Mix in the green chilies, garlic, cardamom seeds, ginger, cinnamon sticks, and cloves.

Cook for about 5 minutes, stirring frequently until the garlic begins to brown.

Stir in the coriander, cumin, garlic powder, and cayenne pepper. Pour in the water and simmer until the mixture has thickened and most of the water has evaporated.

Add the beef to the pressure cooker and coat well with the spice mixture. Pour in the water, close and lock the lid. Cook on high pressure for 40 minutes.

When the cooking time is up, release the pressure using the quick release method. Serve warm.

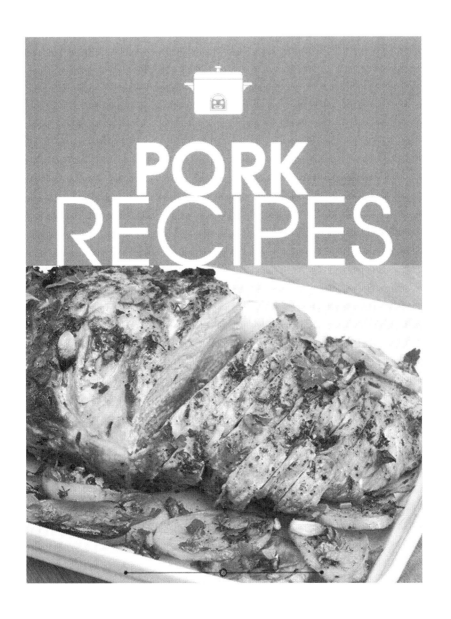

PORK RECIPES

Pressure Cooker Carnitas

Calories: 153

Fats: 8g

Carbs: 3g

Protein: 16g

Sodium: 130mg

Servings: 8-12

Cook time: 1 hour

Ingredients:

3 pounds boneless pork shoulder, cut into 1 ½-inch cubes

3 tablespoons canola oil

2 fresh poblano peppers, roughly chopped

3 jalapeno peppers, roughly chopped

1 serrano pepper, roughly chopped

4 cloves garlic, roughly chopped

1 large onion, roughly chopped

3 teaspoons ground cumin

2 teaspoons ground coriander

1 1/2 cups low sodium beef broth

Directions:

Pour the oil in your pressure cooker over medium-high heat. Add the pork cubes when the oil is hot enough and brown them nicely on all sides.

Mix in the jalapeno, poblano, Serrano peppers, garlic, onion, cumin, coriander, and beef broth.

Close and lock the lid of your pressure cooker. Cook under medium pressure for an hour. When the cooking time is up, use the cold water method to release the pressure. Serve warm.

Pork Chop Casserole

Calories: 250

Fats: 10g

Carbs: 15g

Protein: 16g

Sodium: 130mg

Servings: 4

Cook time: 15 minutes

Ingredients:

4 1-inch pork chops

4 medium potatoes, peeled and thinly sliced

¼ cup homemade chicken stock

1 onion, thinly sliced

¾ cup lemon juice

1 bay leaf, finely crushed

Chopped parsley, to taste

Black pepper

Directions:

Pour the oil in your pressure cooker and heat it.

Sprinkle the pork chops with pepper and salt and add to the pressure cooker. When the pork chops are seared, remove them and keep warm.

Use the chicken broth to deglaze the pressure cooker. This will loosen up the particles stuck to the bottom of the pressure cooker.

Add half of the onions and potatoes in the cooker and sprinkle with black pepper and chopped parsley.

Return the pork chops to the pressure cooker and sprinkle with the crushed bay leaf. Arrange the remaining potato and onion slices on top of the pork chops. Again, sprinkle with black pepper and chopped parsley.

Pour in the water and close and lock the lid. Cook on high pressure for 10 minutes. When the cooking time is up, release the pressure using the natural release method.

Herbed Pork Roast

Calories: 180

Fats: 9g

Carbs: 15g

Protein: 17g

Sodium: 130mg

Servings: 4-6

Cook time: 26 minutes

Ingredients:

1 ½ pounds boneless pork loin

1 tablespoon olive oil

1 garlic cloves, peeled and crushed

3 medium potatoes, diced

1 teaspoon thyme

½ teaspoon basil

1 teaspoon crushed rosemary

½ teaspoon marjoram

½ cup water

Black pepper

Directions:

Season the pork with pepper and press with your palm so that it adheres. Set aside.

Pour the oil in your pressure cooker, and when the oil is hot enough, add the potatoes and brown them until nicely golden. Remove the potatoes from the cooker and set aside.

Add the pork to the pressure cooker and brown it on all sides. Stir in the crushed garlic and cook for one more minute until fragrant.

Sprinkle the pork with the thyme, basil, rosemary, and marjoram. Pour the water around the pork.

Close and lock the lid. Cook on high pressure for 15 minutes. When the cooking time is up, quick release the pressure.

Open the cooker and add the potatoes. Close and lock the lid again. Cook on high pressure for 6 more minutes. When done, quick release the pressure. Serve warm.

Pressure Cooker Pork Tenderloin

Calories: 151

Fats: 10g

Carbs: 3g

Protein: 12g

Sodium: 120mg

Servings: 5

Cook time: 25 min

Ingredients:

¼ cup olive oil

¼ cup fresh cilantro leaves

2 cloves garlic, sliced

¼ cup lime juice

½ teaspoon red pepper flakes, or to taste

1 pound pork tenderloin

¾ cup low sodium chicken broth

¼ cup lemon juice

Directions:

Combine the olive oil, cilantro, garlic, lime juice, and red pepper flakes in a blender. Blend well until smooth. Pour the mixture into a large plastic bag.

Add the pork to the bag with the sauce. Seal the bag and give it a few shakes to make sure that the pork is coated with the marinade. Open the bag and seal it again to remove as much air as possible from the bag. Keep the pork in the fridge for 8 hours.

Combine the broth and lemon juice in your pressure cooker. Place the pork tenderloin in this liquid and add the remaining marinade in the pressure cooker.

Close and lock the lid of your pressure cooker. Cook on medium pressure for 25 minutes. When the cooking time is up, leave the cooker to sit for 5 minutes. Hold the cooker under a stream of cold water to release the pressure.

Remove the tenderloin from the pressure cooker and slice it into medallions. Serve warm.

Peasant Soup

Calories: 164

Fat: 4g

Carbs: 22g

Protein: 12g

Sodium: 28g

Servings: 6

Cook time: 45 minutes

Ingredients:

1 small smoked ham hock

¼ cup finely chopped onion

¼ cup chopped celery

½ cup finely grated carrot

1 cup split peas or lentils, soaked for several hours

4 cups water

1 bay leaf

1 sprig parsley, finely sliced

1/8 teaspoon thyme

Directions:

Combine the ham hock, onion, celery, carrot, and lentils in your pressure cooker. Pour in the water. Mix in the bay leaf, parsley, thyme and season with salt and pepper.

Close and lock the lid. Cook at medium pressure for 45 minutes. When the cooking time is up, use the quick release method to release the pressure.

Remove the ham hock from the pressure cooker, skin it and dice. Add the ham hock dice back to the soup. Serve warm.

SEAFOOD/FISH RECIPES

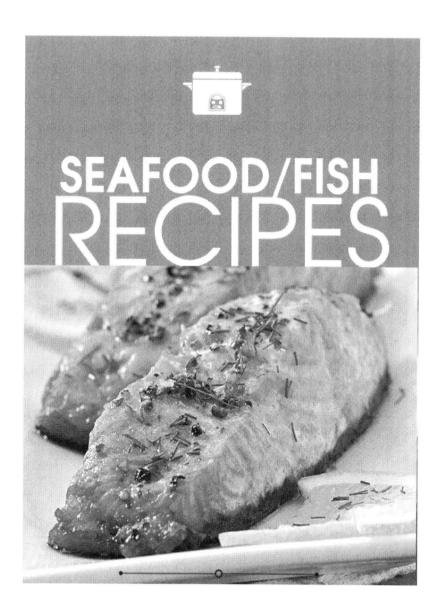

Coconut Fish Curry

Calories: 210

Fat: 6g

Carbs: 12g

Protein: 26.1g

Sodium: 190mg

Servings: 6-8

Cook time: 15 minutes

Ingredients:

Vegetable oil

6 curry leaves

2 garlic cloves, squeezed

2 onions, cut into strips

1 tablespoon freshly grated ginger

2 teaspoons ground cumin

1 tablespoon ground coriander

1 teaspoon hot pepper flakes

1/2 teaspoon ground turmeric

1/2 teaspoon ground fenugreek

2 cups unsweetened coconut milk

1 tomato, chopped

2 capsicums, cut into strips

1 ½ pounds fish fillets, cut into bite-size pieces, rinsed

Lemon juice to taste

Directions:

Preheat your pressure cooker on medium-low heat. Pour some oil and add the curry leaves. Fry the leaves for a minute. Stir in the garlic, onions, and ginger and sauté until the onions gets soft.

Mix in the cumin, coriander, hot pepper, turmeric, and fenugreek. Continue sautéing for 2 more minutes. Pour in the coconut milk to deglaze the base of the cooker. Scrape with a wooden spoon to make sure that nothing sticks to the bottom of the pressure cooker.

Stir in the tomatoes and capsicum and add the fish. Stir well to coat the fish with the sauce mixture.

Close and lock the lid. Cook at low pressure for 5 minutes. When the cooking time is up, release the pressure using the quick release method. Drizzle with the lemon juice and serve.

Potato & Octopus Salad

Calories: 119

Fat: 0g

Carbs: 27g

Protein: 3g

Sodium: 10 mg

Servings: 6-8

Cook time: 50 minutes

Ingredients:

1 (about 2 pounds) octopus

2 pounds potatoes

1 garlic cloves, whole

1 bay leaf

1/2 tablespoon peppercorns

1 bunch parsley, chopped

For the vinaigrette:

½ cup olive oil

4-5 tablespoons white wine vinegar

2 garlic cloves, crushed

Directions:

First, prepare the octopus. Remove its head and then slit it in half. To remove the contents from the inside, turn it inside out. Discard the beak in the center (the place where the tentacles meet). Hold the octopus under a stream of water and rinse it well.

Scrub the potatoes well and place them unpeeled and whole in your pressure cooker. Pour in enough water to cover the potatoes halfway. Close and lock the lid of your pressure cooker. Cook on low pressure for 15 minutes.

Once the cooking time is up, release the pressure using the quick release method and take the potatoes out of the pressure cooker. Don't discard the cooking liquid. Peel the hot potatoes; dice them into small cubes and place in a large mixing bowl.

To cook the octopus in the pressure cooker, pour enough water to almost cover it. Add the bay leaf, whole garlic clove, and peppercorns and bring to the boil. Then add the octopus.

Close and lock the lid. Cook on low pressure for 15 minutes. When the time is up, release the pressure using the quick release method and check the octopus. If the octopus is not fork-tender in the thickest part of its flesh, you can cook it under pressure for a minute or two.

Once the octopus is done, take it out of the pressure cooker and remove any remaining skin. To do that, you can lightly drag a knife over the tentacles. Chop the tentacles and head into small chunks. Add the octopus chunks to the bowl with the potatoes and mix well.

To prepare the vinaigrette, combine all the ingredients in a jar and shake well to blend everything.

Flood the octopus and potato chunks with the vinaigrette, garnish with the chopped parsley and serve.

Almond Cod with Peas

Calories: 210.

Fat: 7g

Carbs: 11g

Protein: 26g

Sodium: 295mg

Servings: 4

Cook time: 30 minutes

Ingredients:

2 tablespoons sliced almonds, divided

1 tablespoon vegetable oil

½ cup lightly packed parsley sprig

2 large garlic cloves, cut in half

½ teaspoon paprika

1 tablespoon fresh oregano sprigs

1 cup water

1 pound frozen cod fish fillet

10 ounces frozen peas

Directions:

First, take the fish out of your freezer and leave it to defrost at room temperature.

Combine the parsley, garlic, one tablespoon almonds, oregano, and paprika in your food processor. Pulse until combined and finely chopped. Set aside.

Pour the oil into your pressure cooker. When the oil is heated, add the remaining almonds and brown them lightly. Remove the almonds, place them on a paper towel and set aside.

Pour the water in the pressure cooker and mix in the herb mixture prepared in the food processor. Insert the steamer basket, slice the fish into four equal pieces and place them in the basket.

Close and lock the lid. Cook on high pressure for two minutes. When the cooking time is up, release the pressure using the cold water release method.

Open the pressure cooker and remove the fish and the basket. Keep the fish warm.

Add the frozen peas to the pressure cooker and close and lock the lid again. Cook on high pressure for a minute. Again release the pressure by holding the pressure cooker under a stream of cold water.

Transfer the peas into a serving dish and top them with the fish slices. Sprinkle with the browned almonds before serving.

Pressure Cooker Salmon Steaks

Calories: 264

Fat: 7g

Carbs: 4g

Protein: 40g

Sodium: 70mg

Servings: 4

Cook time: 29 minutes

Ingredients:

3 pounds salmon steaks

1 teaspoon black pepper

1 medium onion, thinly sliced

1 ½ cups water

1 lemon, thinly sliced

Directions:

Prepare your pressure cooker by placing a trivet inside. Pour in the water.

Season the fish with the pepper and place it on the trivet.

Arrange the lemon and onion slices on top of the fish but reserve a few lemon slices for garnish.

Close and lock the lid. Cook on high pressure for 6 minutes. When the cooking time is up, release the pressure using the quick release method.

Open the cooker, remove the fish and place it on a serving dish.

Discard the lemon and onion slices. Garnish the fish with a few lemon slices and serve hot.

Lemon, Artichoke, and Shrimp Risotto

Calories: 510

Fat: 19g

Carbs: 60g

Protein: 25g

Sodium: 250g

Servings: 4

Cook time: 45 minutes

Ingredients:

3 ¼ cups low sodium chicken broth

2 teaspoons olive oil

½ cup minced onion

1 ½ cups Arborio rice

¼ cup water

14 ounces artichoke hearts, quartered

½ pound large shrimp, defrosted if frozen, peeled and deveined

Freshly ground black pepper, to taste

For the "cheese":

1 cup raw almonds

2 tablespoons nutritional yeast

Directions:

Pour the chicken broth in a pot and warm it over medium heat. Set aside. Add the olive oil into your pressure cooker and heat it. Stir in the minced onion and sauté for 2-3 minutes until soft. Do not brown the onions.

Add the rice and mix well to coat the grains with oil and onion mixture. Leave the rice to toast for a minute.

Pour in the water and cook stirring occasionally until most of the liquid has been absorbed. Add the warm chicken broth.

Close and lock the lid. Cook at high pressure for 6 minutes. When the cooking time is up, release the pressure using the quick release method.

Open the cooker and mix in the lemon zest, artichoke hearts, and shrimp. Stir well to combine the shrimp and artichoke hearts with the rice to allow the heat to cook the shrimp. This will take about 2 minutes.

In the meantime, prepare the cheese. Place all the cheese ingredients in your blender or food processor. Pulse until the mixture gets the desired consistency.

Add the cheese to the risotto and stir well. The cheese and rice will absorb some of the remaining liquid in the risotto. Serve warm.

Citrus Cauliflower Salad with Anchovies

Calories: 170

Fat: 9g

Carbs: 22g

Protein: 4g

Sodium: 210mg

Servings: 6-8

Cook time: 10 minutes

Ingredients:

1 cup water

1 small romanesco cauliflower, divided into florets

1 small cauliflower, divided into florets

1 pound broccoli

2 seedless oranges, peeled and thinly sliced

For the vinaigrette:

1 orange, zested and squeezed

1 hot pepper, sliced or chopped

4 anchovies, chopped

4 tablespoons extra virgin olive oil

Directions:

To prepare the vinaigrette, combine the orange juice and zest, hot pepper, anchovies, and olive oil in a container that can be sealed. Shake the container until the ingredients are well-combined. Set aside.

Pour the water in your pressure cooker. Set the steamer basket and place all the florets inside.

Close and lock the lid. Cook on low pressure for six minutes. When the cooking time is up, release the pressure using the quick release method.

Transfer the steamed florets into a serving dish and mix in the orange slices. Shake the container with the vinaigrette once again and drizzle the florets.
Serve immediately.

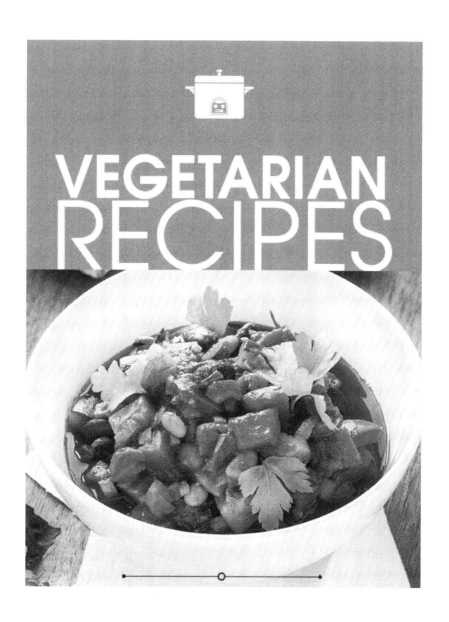

VEGETARIAN
RECIPES

Cinnamon-Scented Breakfast Quinoa

Calories 160

Carbs 28g

Fat 3g

Protein 6g

Sodium 7mg

Servings: 4

Cook time: 30 minutes

Ingredients:

1 cup quinoa

1 1/2 cups water

2 cinnamon sticks

Broken or chopped walnuts, pure maple syrup or honey

Directions:

Add the quinoa to a bowl and wash it in several changes of water until the water is clear. When washing quinoa, rub grains and allow them to settle before you pour off the water.

Use a large fine-mesh sieve to drain the quinoa. Prepare your pressure cooker with a trivet and steaming basket. Place the quinoa and the cinnamon sticks in the basket and pour the water.

Close and lock the lid. Cook at high pressure for 6 minutes. When the cooking time is up, release the pressure using the quick release method.

Fluff the quinoa with a fork and remove the cinnamon sticks. Divide the cooked quinoa among serving bowls and top with maple syrup or honey, and chopped walnuts.

Zucchini-Basil Soup

Calories: 170

Fat: 14g

Carbs: 10 g

Protein: 3 g

Sodium: 29 mg

Servings: 4-6

Cook time: 30 minutes

Ingredients:

2 pounds zucchini, trimmed and cut crosswise into thirds

¾ cup chopped onion

2 garlic cloves, chopped

¼ cup olive oil

4 cups water, divided

1/3 cup packed basil leaves

Directions:

Use a slicer to julienne skin form half of zucchini.
Drain using a sieve. After about 20 minutes, the

zucchini will get wilted. Roughly chop the remaining zucchini.

Pour the oil in your pressure cooker and add the garlic and onion. Sauté for about 5 minutes stirring occasionally.

When the onion gets soft, mix in the chopped zucchini and cook for 5 more minutes, stirring occasionally. Pour in 3 cups of water and add the basil.

Close and lock the lid. Cook on high pressure for about 3 minutes. When the cooking time is up, release the pressure using the quick release method. Leave the soup to cool.

Working in batches, puree the soup in a blender. Pour the remaining cup of water to a small saucepan. Add the julienned zucchini and blanch it for a minute.

Drain it using a sieve. Season the soup with pepper. Serve in bowls garnished with julienned zucchini.

Summer Breakfast Quinoa Bowls

Calories: 263

Fat: 4 g

Carbs: 48 g

Protein: 11 g

Sodium: 94 mg

Servings: 2

Cook time: 10 minutes

Ingredients:

1/3 cup uncooked quinoa, rinsed well

2 teaspoons brown sugar

½ teaspoon vanilla extract

2/3 + ¾ cup low-fat milk

1 small peach, sliced

14 blueberries

12 raspberries

2 teaspoons honey

Directions:

Preheat your pressure cooker. Combine the quinoa, vanilla, 2/3 cup of milk, and brown sugar. Mix well until the sugar has dissolved.

Close and lock the lid. Cook on high pressure for 6 minutes. When the cooking time is up, release the pressure using the natural release method. Fluff with a fork and set aside.

Spray your pressure cooker base with oil. Add the peaches, blueberries, and raspberries and cook for 2-3 minutes to bring out their sweetness. Set aside.

Divide the cooked quinoa among the serving bowls, pour the remaining milk over, and top with peaches. Drizzle with honey and serve.

Easy Vegetarian Pressure Cooker Beans

Calories: 205

Fat: 4g

Carbs: 31g

Protein: 11g

Sodium: 22mg

Servings: 12

Cook time: 30 minutes

Ingredients:

9 cups water

3 cups dried black beans

3 tablespoons olive oil

1 onion, diced

4 cloves garlic, diced

2 teaspoons black mustard seeds

2 teaspoons cumin seeds

1 cup water or as needed

Directions:

Add the beans to a large pot and pour in 9 cups of water. Leave to soak for 8 hours. Drain the beans and rinse them well.

In your pressure cooker, combine the onion, soaked beans, garlic, mustard seeds, cumin seeds and season with salt. Pour in enough water as specified in your pressure cooker's manual.

Close and lock the lid. Cook on high pressure for 30 minutes. When the cooking time is up, release the pressure using the natural release method. Serve warm.

Kidney Bean Curry

Calories: 224

Fat: 56g

Carbs: 34g

Protein: 11g

Sodium: 16mg

Servings: 8

Cook time: 1 hour

Ingredients:

1 large onion, chopped

2 cups dry red kidney beans

4 garlic cloves, chopped

2-inch piece fresh ginger, chopped

2 teaspoons ghee

2 tablespoons vegetable oil

2 dried red chili peppers, broken into pieces

6 whole cloves

1 teaspoon cumin seeds

1 teaspoon ground cumin

1 teaspoon ground turmeric

1 teaspoon ground coriander

2 cups water

2 tomatoes, chopped

2 teaspoons garam masala

1 teaspoon ground red pepper

1 teaspoon white sugar

¼ cup cilantro leaves, chopped

Directions:

Place the beans into a bowl or pot. Pour in enough cool water to cover the beans by several inches. Leave the beans to soak for 8 hours or overnight. Drain and rinse well.

Use a mortar and pestle to combine the garlic, ginger, and onion into a paste.
Pour the oil and ghee in your pressure cooker.

Heat over medium heat and then add the cumin seeds, chili peppers, and whole cloves. Fry in the hot oil until the cumin seeds begin to crack.

Mix in the garlic paste and cook until golden brown. Stir this mix frequently not allowing it to burn.

Season with the cumin, turmeric, and coriander and cook for a few more seconds. Stir in the tomatoes and cook until the tomatoes get tender. Mix in the drained and rinsed kidney beans. Add enough water to cover the contents of the pressure cooker. Add two additional cups of water. Sprinkle with the sugar.

Close and lock the lid of your pressure cooker. Cook on high pressure for 40 minutes. After this, reduce the heat to low and cook for about 15 more minutes.

When the cooking time is up, release the pressure using the quick release method or leave the pressure to release naturally.

Open your pressure cooker and mix in the ground red pepper and garam masala. Stir well and garnish with chopped cilantro before serving.

Creamy Sweet Potato Soup

Calories: 120

Fat: 0g

Carbs: 25g

Protein: 5g

Sodium: 60mg

Servings: 6-8

Cook time: 10 minutes

Ingredients:

½ cup dried white beans, soaked overnight, drained and rinsed well

1 small yellow onion, chopped

2 medium sweet potatoes, peeled and diced

2 stalks celery, chopped

1 bay leaf

1 tablespoon chopped fresh rosemary

1 tablespoon chopped fresh sage

Directions:

Combine all the ingredients in your pressure cooker. Pour in the amount of water specified in your pressure cooker manual. The cooker should not be filled more than half.

Close and lock the lid. Cook on high pressure for 10 minutes. When the cooking time is up, release the pressure using the natural release method. Open the cooker and discard the bay leaf.

Leave the soup to cool. Working in batches, puree the contents of the pressure cooker in a blender or use an immersion blender. Warm the soup before serving.

Conclusion

Here, you will find delicious recipes that you can prepare in a snap and that follow the DASH diet principles. There's a variety of recipes you can choose from – chicken, beef, pork, seafood/fish, and vegetarian pressure cooker meals. The ingredients are the ones you probably already have in your kitchen.

So, choose a recipe, get the ingredients, throw them in your pressure cooker and that's it. In just several minutes, you will have a tasty and flavorful meal that will provide you with the necessary nutrients your body needs and will, at the same time, keep you away from sodium that can have many negative effects on your health. Choose wisely and use the food to your benefit.

23856636R00049

Printed in Poland
by Amazon Fulfillment
Poland Sp. z o.o., Wrocław